WHY DIVINE HEALING

Amb Promise Ogbonna

WHY DIVINE HEALING

Copyright © January 2020 by Amb Promise Ogbonna

Published by Amb Promise Ogbonna

Unless otherwise indicated, all Scriptural quotations are from the New King James Version

Write Amb Promise Ogbonna

Author and Publisher:

Ontop Life Publishers Company

Send Amb Promise Ogbonna a mail at: info@heavenow.org

Visit Amb. Promise Ogbonna's Website: https://heavenow.org

E-mail: ontoplifepublishers@gmail.com

Tel: +234 8060638053, +234 8053995257, +234 8027829586

CONTENTS

WHY I WROTE THIS BOOK!

I am sent to Publish All the Words of God's Heavenly Kingdom Life for the Restoration of all.

I am not writing human philosophy. I am not writing as a hobby neither am I writing to entertain but to bring Spiritual light, impart, Spiritual, Wisdom and Power to build your faith and transform your life! I have a Mandate from The Lord Jesus Christ to write and these Words are published to meet man's needs in every area of life! This Book, therefore, is published in obedience to the Command of the Lord to make His Words of Life and Wisdom, Solutions and Power available to address every aspect of human needs.

I can say as Paul wrote "My message and my preaching were not in the persuasive language of philosophy, but in demonstration of the Spirit and of power; in order that your faith should rest, not on human philosophy, but on the power of God." 1Corinthians 2:4-5 (BBE)

"For the Kingdom of God is based, not on words, but on power." 1Corinthians 4:20 (BBE)

The Life Publishing Mandate

The Lord sent me to Publish All The Words of His Heavenly Kingdom Life for ALL mankind!

Jesus' last words is to Preach and Publish the Goodnews with proofs to every creature and among all nations (Mark 13:10; 16:15; Matthew 24:14).

The Lord gave us the Goodnews to publish and spread among all nations (Psalm 68:11; Mark 13:10).

In the Book of Esther, the enemy wrote and spread the words of death worldwide to destroy God's people and souls that God loves. [See Esther 3].

But at the command of the king, a new decree and words of life were written and spread to reach everyone (every creature) everywhere that the first words of death had reached. [See Esther 8].

This is our task. We have been given the New Covenant, Heavenly Kingdom, Words of Life to publish and spread to reach every creature everywhere worldwide. The Goodnews is that no one needs to die again! The old decree has been changed. Everyone can now live and enjoy peace and prosperity where each lives. That is why Ontop Mission Life Publishers Company. We are Publishing, Spreading and Bringing the Gospel of Christ and All the Words of life to every creature everywhere.

I will like to share some of the encounters with the Lord Jesus Christ that gave birth to The Life Publishing Mandate and why this Book and my other books:

1. On 2-5-95, Jesus Christ and I stood on the balcony of a great beautiful mansion in Heaven whose foundation I couldn't see (see Amos 9:6). He showed me Preachers, driven by selfishness and being used by the enemy, walking on people's heads and shoulders as their platform to preach. The people were hungry, thirsty, weeping, trampled upon and yet yearning for the TRUTH (see Amos 8:11-13). I saw My Lord shaking His head in disgust. He also brought to my view those in hell and I saw their agony and pain and what a sight it was! Afterward, as we beheld the abuse of His people, He pointed His right hand towards them and said to me, "See what is happening to the people I died for. "The Lord Jesus gave me A WELL USED COPY OF THE BIBLE and said to me "GO and tell them (The Preachers and The People) to Repent and Believe The Gospel Only and they will be Restored." I asked 'How

will I do it? And He said to me, "BE SEPARATE! Go, I send YOU as My Ambassador and Witness with My Authority and Power: Publish The Word, Stop anything after their destruction, Raise, Build and Plant them as My Ambassadors. Let them know the truth. Teach All The TRUTH and Spread them as My Seed ALL over the earth and restore all things."

2. On 6-7-96, The Lord Jesus Christ came to me again and said, "It is well" and gave me a copy of THE BIBLE and said to me, "Take: This is My Staff of Office" – My Authority and Power. After The LORD gave me His Staff of Office [The Word], I saw something like a mist or cloud appear out of the Word and as I watched, a horse emerged from 'within the mist' and jumped about and stopped. The Lord told me The Word is creative and created the horse and is My Rod for working Miracles, Wonders and Signs. I am to Go with it to all, as Moses went with his ROD, and "Stop anything after man's destruction, Bring Healing, Liberty and Restoration to all; Raise, Build and Plant Christ's Ambassadors everywhere and Restore all things."

3. On 20-5-97, I was given a BIBLE and 2 BIROS by Arch. Benson A. Idahosa in a conference that took place in a place like a stadium. And he said to me, "Go and Proclaim and Publish The Everlasting Gospel of Jesus Christ worldwide and deliver the full benefits to all. This Gospel of The Kingdom must be preached in all the world for a witness unto all nations!

4. On 18-11-03, The Lord spoke to me again ON WRITING, and said to me "Write all the hidden mysteries I show you and I will ensure it gets to all the Nations. Prophetic writings is what unveils, reveals, makes known the revelation of the mystery hidden for ages long past. The surest way of unveiling the Gospel and proclaiming Jesus Christ the Lord, is through prophetic writings as God commanded so that all nations will believe and obey God.

5. On 26-11-03, The Lord spoke to me saying, "Write what people can read and understand. It's most important. Your writing must be readable and understandable. Write in such a way that a primary school pupil can read and understand My Words. "The common people heard me gladly." Everyone must read and

understand My Words that you write.

6. On 2-10-04, The Lord Jesus explained to me the vision of 2one fifths s /95 where I Stood with Him on the Balcony of the Mansion in Heaven and He showed me Preachers using the shoulders and heads of people as their platform to preach. They were hungry, thirsty and trampled underfoot yet yearning for the reality. And The Lord commanded me to WRITE and publish His Words for the downtrodden and for all."

7. On10-12-04, The Lord said to me "Write in a book all the Words that I have spoken to you" and He gave me Jeremiah 30:2.

8. On 04-04-05, The Lord said to me "Publish the Word and bring healing, liberty and restoration to all everywhere." See Psalm 68:11 and Psalm 107:20.

9. On 23-12-05, The Lord said to me: Publish The Words, Publish The Works, Publish The Wonders, Make My Deeds Known, and Let Everyone See My Glory Everywhere.

10. On 01-03-13, The Holy Ghost said to me:
Publish the Works of Jesus Christ everywhere
Advertise the Doings of Jesus Christ the Lord.
Make known the Miracles of Jesus Christ the Lord.
Bind the Testimony of the Acts of the Lord Jesus Christ's
Be My Witness of all My Signs and Wonders everywhere.
Share Testimonies of All I AM Doing forever.
Go and Tell All everywhere of All My Miracles and Wonders and Signs and All I have done and commanded you.

The Lord said to me "All who believe that I sent you and receive you as My Ambassador and receive your Words as My Words will experience all the Father sent me to make available to humanity!"

Like Peter, I can tell you "We have not followed cunningly devised fables, when we made known unto you the power and coming of our Lord Jesus Christ, but were eyewitnesses of his majesty." 2Peter 1:16

Beloved, every Word written in this Book is from The Lord and are His Wisdom and Heaven's Solutions packaged and released to deal with your challenges, solve your problems and meet your needs.

Read with an open heart, Believe and Receive The Truth and Pick the Lessons and engage them.

I know you will experience The One who is The Author, Perfecter and Finisher of your faith and Who is The Real Author of this Book. He is Jesus Christ, The Son of The Living God. And He is the Same yesterday and today and forever!

"O LORD, how manifold are Your works! In wisdom You have made them all. The earth is full of Your possessions." Psalm 104:24

I guarantee you that you will never be the same again as you embrace God's Wisdom in This Book!

God Bless you.

Your brother and His Steward for the benefit of all,

Ambassador Promise Ogbonna

THE HEAVENLY MANDATE & VISION

The Heavenly Mandate

To Preach The Everlasting Gospel to Everyone everywhere, Stop anything after man's destruction, Bring Healing, Liberty and Restoration to ALL; Raise, Build and Plant All as Christ's Ambassadors on His Living Mission everywhere and Restore all things!

The Heavenly Vision

To Restore All Things Everywhere at All Cost and By All Means! Acts 3:21

FIRST WORDS

Ninety five percent of the world's population of over 7.7 billion people as at April 2019, are sick! Majority of them are sick because they don't understand the reason Why God Heals and so have failed to take advantage of it!

God is The ONLY Wise God and when His wisdom is trivialized or not sought the result is always adverse. The reason Why God heals has not been made clear to the sick therefore, billions of the sick have remained sick and many have died sick due to their ignorance.

Healing is the first thing God always does to make man and restore him to God's image and likeness. God is so eager to the sick that He sent His only begotten Son Jesus The Christ to take the stripes required to free every human being alive on earth today from every sickness and every disease.

But though God is so eager to heal all the sick, He does not want to waste His provision on those that will trample it underfoot. For when purpose is not clear, abuse is always inevitable.

God says "Give not that which is holy unto the dogs, neither cast ye your pearls before swine, lest they trample them under their feet, and turn again and rend you." Matthew 7:6. God does not want waste His Healing on those who will waste it. God's healing is costly, very costly yet free!

Therefore, this Book! It presents to humanity WHY DIVINE HEALING. It shows Why God Heals!

Please, don't toy with what you are about read in this Book.

This is God's heartbeat unveiled. It will place within your reach what you need to be free from sickness and disease and live in health the remaining days of your life as God wants, doing what He wants..

Read and Arise and Shine! Its Your Moment of Glory. Peace!

CHAPTER 1

WHY DIVINE HEALING

It is God's only solution to your suffering.

It is God's only provision to permanently keep you out of sickness/disease.

Ecclesiastes 3:14

"I know that, whatsoever God doeth, it shall be forever: nothing can be put to it, nor any thing taken from it: and God doeth it, that men should fear before him."

Whatever God does is forever. Nothing can be added to it and nothing can be taken from it, because God has done/does it so that men should fear before him.

Nothing man does is forever.

Man's provisions are not forever.

Man's gifts are not forever.

Man's "healings" are not forever.

Man's prosperity is not forever.

Man's solutions to your problems doesn't last forever.

Man's work to help you of your challenges does not last forever.

If man "heals" you today, be sure that you will still have the same ailment again and again.

My wife's Aunt was operated more than twice on the same breast for the same sickness.

A lady I know (Ify) told me she was operated 3 times on the same case, for the same reason, by the same doctor. Yet she wasn't healed.

A girl in a church I attended died of cancer after her leg was amputated because the cancer could not be cut off but grew again.

I have seen that vain is the help of man even as God says.

Nothing a man does lasts forever.

But whatever the Lord does lasts forever because He upholds it by Himself with His own power. (Ecclesiastes 3:14; Hebrews 1:3).

This is why I know that your Healing today will be forever if only you believe.

Matthew 8:17

"That it might be fulfilled which was spoken by Isaiah the prophet, saying: "He Himself took our infirmities and bore our sicknesses."

Isaiah 53:4-5

4 "Surely He has borne our griefs And carried our sorrows; Yet we esteemed Him stricken, Smitten by God, and afflicted.

5 But He was wounded for our transgressions, He was bruised for our iniquities; The chastisement for our peace was upon Him, And by His stripes we are healed."

1Peter 2:24

"Who Himself bore our sins in His own body on the tree, that we, having died to sins, might live for righteousness--by whose stripes you were healed."

Psalms 107:20

"He sent His word and healed them, And delivered them from their destructions."

Hebrews 4:12

"For the word of God is living and powerful, and sharper than any two-edged sword, piercing even to the division of soul and spirit, and of joints and marrow, and is a discerner of the thoughts and intents of the heart."

Proverbs 4:22

"For they are life to those who find them, And health to all their flesh."

Ecclesiastes 3:14

"I know that whatever God does, It shall be forever. Nothing can be added to it, And nothing taken from it. God does it, that men should fear before Him."

Exodus 15:26

"And said, "If you diligently heed the voice of the LORD your God and do what is right in His sight, give ear to His commandments and keep all His statutes, I will put none of the diseases on you which I have brought on the Egyptians. For I am the LORD who heals you."

Exodus 13:8

"And you shall tell your son in that day, saying, 'This is done because of what the LORD did for me when I came up from Egypt.'

SICKNESS IS NEVER GOD'S WILL FOR MAN (YOU).

God did not make man sick in the beginning. Man can help you to prolong your suffering if you have, Cancer, HIV/AIDS etc. But if you will allow God, He'll step in Today and now and He'll take care of your sickness and once he does, that will be the last you'll ever see it.

Acts 10:38

"How God anointed Jesus of Nazareth with the Holy Spirit and with power, who went about doing good and healing all who were oppressed by the devil, for God was with Him."

1John 3:8

"He who sins is of the devil, for the devil has sinned from the beginning. For this purpose, the Son of God was manifested, that He might destroy the works of the devil."

Hebrews 13:8

"Jesus Christ is the same yesterday, today, and forever."

Malachi 3:6

"For I am the LORD, I do not change; Therefore, you are not consumed, O sons of Jacob."

John 17:18

"As You sent Me into the world, I also have sent them into the world."

John 20:21

"So, Jesus said to them again, "Peace to you! As the Father has sent Me, I also send you."

John 14:12

"So, Jesus said to them again, "Peace to you! As the Father has sent Me, I also send you."

Proverb 13:17

"A wicked messenger falls into trouble, but a faithful ambassador brings health."

You cannot be abandoned in your suffering. That's why He sent me as the Father sent Him and He is now here with me. That's why I know there is no manner of sickness nor disease that will be left in your body.

Proverbs 13:17

"A wicked messenger falls into mischief: but a faithful ambassador is health."

John 14:12

"Verily, verily, I say unto you, He that believeth on me, the works that I do shall he do also; and greater works than these shall he do; because I go unto my Father."

Matthew 9:35

"Then Jesus went about all the cities and villages, teaching in their synagogues, preaching the gospel of the kingdom, and healing every sickness and every disease among the people."

Matthew 4:23-25

23 "And Jesus went about all Galilee, teaching in their synagogues, preaching the gospel of the kingdom, and healing all kinds of sickness and all kinds of disease among the people.

24 Then His fame went throughout all Syria; and they brought to Him all sick people who were afflicted with various diseases and torments, and those who were demon-possessed, epileptics, and paralytics; and He healed them.

25 Great multitudes followed Him--from Galilee, and from Decapolis, Jerusalem, Judea, and beyond the Jordan."

I am here to stop whatever is after your destructions.

THE LIVING COMMISSION: The Time Is Up! Heal Them and Stop Anything After Their Destructions, Raise, Build, And Plant

My Ambassadors for Me Worldwide, Go! I Have Sent You to Accomplish This Task!

THE LIVING MISSION: To Heal All and Stop Anything After Their Destructions; Raise, Build, and plant Christ's Ambassadors Worldwide in This Generation.

THE LIVING VISSION: World Emancipation and Final Recovery of All Things at All Cost and By All Means.

The Time is up! Therefore, the enemy afflicting your bodies, soul and spirit must stop all their evil works now in Jesus Name.

I command them to stop now.

I proclaim/announce your healing/deliverance now in Jesus Name. Be healed. Be free, be delivered. Be loosed now in Jesus Name.

WHY DIVINE HEALING OR REASONS FOR DIVINE HEALING.

According to Scriptures, the fundamental reason Why God Heals or for Divine Healing is to fulfill God's plan and agenda in Genesis 1:26-28. "Then God said, "Let Us make man in Our image, according to Our likeness; let them have dominion over the fish of the sea, over the birds of the air, and over the cattle, over all the earth and over every creeping thing that creeps on the earth. So, God created man in His own image; in the image of God He created him; male and female He created them. Then God blessed them, and God said to them, "Be fruitful and multiply; fill the earth and subdue it; have dominion over the fish of the sea, over the birds of the air, and over every living thing that moves on the earth."

God wants man to be free from sickness and disease and live as healthy as God lives so that man can take his place in God's plan here on earth. It takes ONLY MAN'S DIVINE HEALTH spirit, and soul and body for him to live and fulfill God's divine agenda for man. This is the foundational pillar why God Heals and those who don't know it nor comply with it will struggle to receive healing from God and may still not be able to. God hates wasting His provisions.

Below are other reasons Why Divine Healing:

1. To Bring Jesus into every life or soul and into every family, Luke 10:1-3

1 "After these things the Lord appointed seventy others also, and sent them two by two before His face into every city and place where He Himself was about to go.

2 Then He said to them, "The harvest truly is great, but the laborers are few; therefore, pray the Lord of the harvest to send out laborers into His harvest.

3 "Go your way; behold, I send you out as lambs among wolves."

It is God's plan to Raise and Recover the lost.

2. It is to do good to all who free all under the oppression of the devil. Acts 10:38

"How God anointed Jesus of Nazareth with the Holy Spirit and with power, who went about doing good and healing all who were oppressed by the devil, for God was with Him."

Luke 4:14,37

14 "Then Jesus returned in the power of the Spirit to Galilee, and news of Him went out through all the surrounding region.

37 And the report about Him went out into every place in the surrounding region."

Mark 1:33

"And the whole city was gathered together at the door."

Matthew 4:23-25

23 "And Jesus went about all Galilee, teaching in their synagogues, preaching the gospel of the kingdom, and healing all kinds of sickness and all kinds of disease among the people.

24 Then His fame went throughout all Syria; and they brought to Him all sick people who were afflicted with various diseases and torments, and those who were demon-possessed, epileptics, and paralytics; and He healed them.

25 Great multitudes followed Him--from Galilee, and from Decapolis, Jerusalem, Judea, and beyond the Jordan."

It is our advertisement package/tool for escape from obscurity.

3. To free the broken hearted and restore jubilee to every life. Luke 4:18.

The major cause of broken-heartedness is disappointment. He sent me to stop your disappointment, give you new appointment.

Isaiah 61:1-5

1 "The Spirit of the Lord GOD is upon Me, Because the LORD has anointed Me To preach good tidings to the poor; He has sent Me to heal the brokenhearted, to proclaim liberty to the captives, And the opening of the prison to those who are bound;

2 To proclaim the acceptable year of the LORD, And the day of vengeance of our God; To comfort all who mourn,

3 To console those who mourn in Zion, to give them beauty for ashes, the oil of joy for mourning, the garment of praise for the spirit of heaviness; That they may be called trees of righteousness, the planting of the LORD, that He may be glorified."

4 And they shall rebuild the old ruins, they shall raise up the former desolations, and they shall repair the ruined cities, The desolations of many generations.

5 Strangers shall stand and feed your flocks, And the sons of the foreigner Shall be your plowmen and your vinedressers."

Man's hurt cannot be healed by drugs, an operation, psychologists, psychiatrists, Doctors, etc. only Jesus can heal you and you remain healed. That's why Divine Healing and why He sent me. All you need is a touch from the Lord!

Inner wounds e.g. Hurts, Disappointments are more incurable than cancer, HIV, etc; but Jesus has sent me to heal and free you all from all of these.

4. Divine Healing makes the Christ's Ambassadors relevant. Without Divine Healing, the Ambassadors is Irrelevant because anything else we do can be done well-even better by the world of unbelievers.

Divine Healing only makes us relevant, not our teaching/ preaching. We don't have orators/phonetic speakers. We are not meant to be that much. We are to be men of power who control the unseen realms.

The dying, hungry, hurting, poor world needs God not empty words/ideas or opinions. They need the most powerful God for it is only God that can help man, not grammar.

1Corinthians 2:1-5,9-12

1 "And I, brethren, when I came to you, did not come with excellence of speech or of wisdom declaring to you the testimony of God.

2 For I determined not to know anything among you except Jesus Christ and Him crucified.

3 I was with you in weakness, in fear, and in much trembling.

4 And my speech and my preaching were not with persuasive words of human wisdom, but in demonstration of the Spirit and of power,

5 that your faith should not be in the wisdom of men but in the power of God."

1 Corinthians 4:20

"For the kingdom of God is not in word but in power."

Romans 15:17-20

17 "Therefore I have reason to glory in Christ Jesus in the things which pertain to God.

18 For I will not dare to speak of any of those things which Christ has not accomplished through me, in word and deed, to make the Gentiles obedient--

19 in mighty signs and wonders, by the power of the Spirit of God, so that from Jerusalem and round about to Illyricum I have fully preached the gospel of Christ.

20 And so I have made it my aim to preach the gospel, not where Christ was named, lest I should build on another man's foundation,"

2 Corinthians 12:12

"Truly the signs of an apostle were accomplished among you with all perseverance, in signs and wonders and mighty deeds."

Hebrews 2:4

"God also bearing witness both with signs and wonders, with various miracles, and gifts of the Holy Spirit, according to His own will?"

Acts 10:38

"How God anointed Jesus of Nazareth with the Holy Spirit and with power, who went about doing good and healing all who were oppressed by the devil, for God was with Him."

Acts 2:22

"Men of Israel, hear these words: Jesus of Nazareth, a Man attested by God to you by miracles, wonders, and signs which God did through Him in your midst, as you yourselves also know."

We are Irrelevant without Divine Healing.

We are Replaceable without Divine Healing.

We are obsolete without Divine Healing. (The world is ahead in technology)

We are fakes without Divine Healing.

We are wasters without Divine Healing.

We are a Disappointment without divine Healing.

We are noisemakers without Divine Healing.

We are Deceivers without Divine Healing.

We are whited sepulcher without Divine Healing.

We are unimportant without Divine Healing.

We are a mockery of ourselves without Divine Healing.

I am not an ORATOR; I don't want to be.

I am an ORACLE-GOD'S ORACLE. AN ORACLE OF DEITY and I am glad about it and will ever remain AN ORACLE.

I have something to offer my Generation from the LORD of Hosts. He is the one that sent me.

I represent Him. I am His Ambassador. I am here because He wants me here and there is nothing the enemy can do about it. I am absolutely loaded here because I am relevant. I must offer to you all He sent me to give to you.

He has all the answers/solutions to every of your life challenges and He sent me as His channel for the release of such to you and to humanity.

I matter to God, heaven, the earth/world and you. For your sake He sent me. You must receive what He sent me to give to you.

No Government/man can give what He sent me to offer you. I cannot be replaced. I am Relevant. I will fulfill my purpose-unfailingly in Jesus Name.

The Government/Teachers/Medical Doctors, etc cannot give what He sent me to give to you. I am unique and my place no other can take.

-The Government is to provide schools, Hospitals, etc. we are only providing same to Heal the School system/Health system because they are sick. Every facet of our lives that is sick needs Divine Healing and we are here to provide Divine Healing to every area of man's life/Endeavour.

Jesus Christ is the Saviour of man. We want to offer Him to the world. He's The Living Word- Spirit/life (John 1:1-3; 6:63).

5. Divine Healing is for the captives to be free. Alcoholics/ Adulteress/fornicators, drug addicts, Homosexuals, Lesbians, Masturbators, etc can only be set free by the power of the Holy Spirit via Divine Health.

A snake was inserted into a woman because she wanted children. Divine Health will terminate your bareness and give you children. Occultic powers are destroyed and victims are set free via Divine Healing.

God chose my Profession (Preaching) as the greatest/Best profession to help mankind and pays the highest to me-even when He came, He came only to practice my Profession.

If Jesus could have helped the world better being a Carpenter, Medical Doctor, Banker, etc, He could have come as one. But He was sent to destroy the works of the devil via Preaching the Living Word- Teaching, preaching and healing (Matthew 4:23-25; Luke 4:18-19; Isaiah 61:1-4).

Prophet Elisha healed the sick water-2Kings 2:19-22.

Pray/Praise/Believe God/speak boldly for more miracles.

6. Divine Healing is needed because we can only be healed and kept in Divine Health via God's power.

Jeremiah 17:14

"Heal me, O LORD, and I shall be healed; Save me, and I shall be saved, For You are my praise."

Proverbs 4:22

"For they are life to those who find them, And health to all their flesh."

1Thessalonians 5:23

"Now may the God of peace Himself sanctify you completely; and may your whole spirit, soul, and body be preserved blameless at the coming of our Lord Jesus Christ."

7. Jesus dominates all evil forces/Satan because of the Divine Healings and so can we.

Luke 4:18-19,40-41

18 "The Spirit of the LORD is upon Me, Because He has anointed Me To preach the gospel to the poor; He has sent Me to heal the brokenhearted, to proclaim liberty to the captives and recovery of sight to the blind, to set at liberty those who are oppressed;

19 To proclaim the acceptable year of the LORD."

40 When the sun was setting, all those who had any that were sick with various diseases brought them to Him; and He laid His hands on every one of them and healed them.

41 And demons also came out of many, crying out and saying, "You are the Christ, the Son of God!" And He, rebuking them, did not allow them to speak, for they knew that He was the Christ."

We are going to save/recover all by Divine Healing.

8. Divine Healing establishes The Kingdom of God.

Luke 10:9,17

9 "And heal the sick there, and say to them, 'The kingdom of God has come near to you.'

17 Then the seventy returned with joy, saying, "Lord, even the demons are subject to us in Your name."

Matthew 10:1

"And when He had called His twelve disciples to Him, He gave them power over unclean spirits, to cast them out, and to heal all kinds of sickness and all kinds of disease."

Luke 9:1,6

1 "Then He called His twelve disciples together and gave them power and authority over all demons, and to cure diseases.

6 So they departed and went through the towns, preaching the gospel and healing everywhere."

9. Divine Healing brings Joy.

Psalms 16:9-11

9 "Therefore my heart is glad, and my glory rejoices; My flesh also will rest in hope.

10 For You will not leave my soul in Sheol, nor will You allow

Your Holy One to see corruption.

11 You will show me the path of life; In Your presence is fullness of joy; At Your right hand are pleasures forevermore."

John 16:23-24

23 "And in that day you will ask Me nothing. Most assuredly, I say to you, whatever you ask the Father in My name He will give you.

24 "Until now you have asked nothing in My name. Ask, and you will receive, that your joy may be full."

Jeremiah 17:14

"Heal me, O LORD, and I shall be healed; Save me, and I shall be saved, For You are my praise."

10. Divine Healing is God's channel of extending the influence of ministers.

John 17:18

"As You sent Me into the world, I also have sent them into the world."

John 14:12

"Most assuredly, I say to you, he who believes in Me, the works that I do he will do also; and greater works than these he will do, because I go to My Father."

Genesis 1:28

"Then God blessed them, and God said to them, "Be fruitful and multiply; fill the earth and subdue it; have dominion over the fish of the sea, over the birds of the air, and over every living thing that moves on the earth."

Proverbs 13:17

"A wicked messenger falls into trouble, but a faithful ambassador brings health."

11. Divine Healing humbles the proud of this world and subdues almost all oppositions.

Luke 13:31-32

"On that very day some Pharisees came, saying to Him, "Get out and depart from here, for Herod wants to kill You."

John 12:17-19

17 "Therefore the people, who were with Him when He called

Lazarus out of his tomb and raised him from the dead, bore witness.

18 For this reason the people also met Him, because they heard that He had done this sign.

19 The Pharisees therefore said among themselves, "You see that you are accomplishing nothing. Look, the world has gone after Him!"

12. Divine Healing opens up every aspect of our ministry and brings glory/honour to God.

John 11:40-44

40 "Jesus said to her, "Did I not say to you that if you would believe you would see the glory of God?"

41 Then they took away the stone from the place where the dead man was lying. And Jesus lifted up His eyes and said, "Father, I thank You that You have heard Me."

Luke 13:10-18

10 "Now He was teaching in one of the synagogues on the Sabbath.

11 And behold, there was a woman who had a spirit of infirmity eighteen years, and was bent over and could in no way raise herself up.

12 But when Jesus saw her, He called her to Him and said to her, "Woman, you are loosed from your infirmity."

13 And He laid His hands on her, and immediately she was made straight, and glorified God.

14 But the ruler of the synagogue answered with indignation, because Jesus had healed on the Sabbath; and he said to the crowd, "There are six days on which men ought to work; therefore, come and be healed on them, and not on the Sabbath day."

15 The Lord then answered him and said, "Hypocrite! Does not each one of you on the Sabbath lose his ox or donkey from the stall, and lead it away to water it?

16 "So ought not this woman, being a daughter of Abraham, whom Satan has bound--think of it--for eighteen years, be loosed from this bond on the Sabbath?"

17 And when He said these things, all His adversaries were put

to shame; and all the multitude rejoiced for all the glorious things that were done by Him.

18 Then He said, "What is the kingdom of God like? And to what shall I compare it?"

Isaiah 11:9

"There shall come forth a Rod from the stem of Jesse, and a Branch shall grow out of his roots."

Habakkuk 2:14

"For the earth will be filled with the knowledge of the glory of the LORD, As the waters cover the sea."

13. Divine Healing draws us closer to God and makes us go deeper with Him.

Everyone Jesus Christ healed followed Him glorifying the Lord God Almighty.

CHAPTER 2

Isaiah 53:4-5

4 "Surely He has borne our griefs and carried our sorrows; Yet we esteemed Him stricken, Smitten by God, and afflicted.

5 But He was wounded for our transgressions, He was bruised for our iniquities; The chastisement for our peace was upon Him, And by His stripes we are healed."

Matthew 8:16-17

16 "When evening had come, they brought to Him many who were demon-possessed. And He cast out the spirits with a word, and healed all who were sick,

17 that it might be fulfilled which was spoken by Isaiah the prophet, saying: "He Himself took our infirmities and bore our sicknesses."

Is taking on CREDIT the goods/Purchases before the payment is made.

It was done 700 years before Jesus Christ fulfilled it. The Israelites took the purchase of the goods (healing) and enjoyed it before ever Christ fulfilled/paid for it, the same way Americans buy and enjoy their products before they make full payment. When(ever) sin goes, Disease and sickness/poverty has to go also! Both came in together. Both have to leave together too.

Matthew 8:16-17

16 "When evening had come, they brought to Him many who were demon-possessed. And He cast out the spirits with a word, and healed all who were sick,

17 that it might be fulfilled which was spoken by Isaiah the prophet, saying: "He Himself took our infirmities and bore our sicknesses."

1Peter 2:24

"Who Himself bore our sins in His own body on the tree, that we, having died to sins, might live for righteousness--by whose stripes you were healed."

Jesus came and paid fully for our sins/sicknesses/diseases. Now there is nothing that should stop us from enjoying the purchased goods (healing/health/prosperity/etc). But because of ignorance, so many of God's people are yet to begin the enjoyment of their purchased/paid for healings/health/prosperity, etc.

For Israel, their healing was purchased on credit and they enjoyed. For us (Galatians 6:16) our healing was paid for and purchased in ADVANCE. Why must we not really enjoy it?

CATEGORIES OF PEOPLE HE WILL HEAL.

1.-The Sick-All of them.

2.-All types/kinds of sicknesses/diseases.

3.-He will heal wounds. "For I will restore health to you and heal you of your wounds,' says the LORD, 'Because they called you an outcast saying: "This is Zion; No one seeks her."' Jeremiah 30:17

4.-He will bind us up-operatable diseases/sowing.

"Come, and let us return to the LORD; For He has torn, but He will heal us; He has stricken, but He will bind us up." Hosea 6:1

Isaiah 30:26.

"Moreover, the light of the moon will be as the light of the sun, And the light of the sun will be sevenfold, As the light of seven days, In the day that the LORD binds up the bruise of His people and heals the stroke of their wound."

5.-Heal your flesh.

Proverbs 3:7-8

7"Do not be wise in your own eyes; Fear the LORD and depart from evil.

8 It will be health to your flesh, And strength to your bones."
Romans 8:11.

"But if the Spirit of Him who raised Jesus from the dead dwells in you, He who raised Christ from the dead will also give life to your mortal bodies through His Spirit who dwells in you."

6.-Heal all tormented by evil spirits.

"Then His fame went throughout all Syria; and they brought to Him all sick people who were afflicted with various diseases and torments, and those who were demon-possessed, epileptics, and paralytics; and He healed them." Matthew 4:24

"Also, a multitude gathered from the surrounding cities to Jerusalem, bringing sick people and those who were tormented by unclean spirits, and they were all healed." Acts 5:16.

7.-The Blind, the lame, the leper, the deaf, the paralyzed, the epileptic, etc.

"The blind see and the lame walk; the lepers are cleansed and the deaf hear; the dead are raised up and the poor have the gospel preached to them." Matthew 11:5

"Then His fame went throughout all Syria; and they brought to Him all sick people who were afflicted with various diseases and torments, and those who were demon-possessed, epileptics, and paralytics; and He healed them." Matthew 4:24

"For unclean spirits, crying with a loud voice, came out of many who were possessed; and many who were paralyzed and lame were healed." Acts 8:7

8.-Healing of pains.

"And God will wipe away every tear from their eyes; there shall be no more death, nor sorrow, nor crying. There shall be no more pain, for the former things have passed away." Revelation 21:4

"For they are life to those who find them, And health to all their flesh." Proverbs 4:22

9.-All your flesh-Brain, eyes, ears, arteries, nerves, veins, heart, lungs, glands, stomach, liver, intestines, kidneys, muscles, bones, flesh, hands, legs, toes, hair, fingers, tongue, mouth, head, body-every part of you.

"No evil shall befall you, nor shall any plague come near your dwelling;" Psalms 91:10

The real you dwells/lives in a house. There shall no plague come nigh thy dwelling (body/house).

Psalms 105:37

"He also brought them out with silver and gold, and there was none feeble among His tribes."

Exodus 11:7

"But against none of the children of Israel shall a dog move its tongue, against man or beast, that you may know that the LORD does make a difference between the Egyptians and Israel."

Exodus 15:26

and said, "If you diligently heed the voice of the LORD your God and do what is right in His sight, give ear to His commandments and keep all His statutes, I will put none of the diseases on you which I have brought on the Egyptians. For I am the LORD who heals you."

Exodus 12:13

'Now the blood shall be a sign for you on the houses where you are. And when I see the blood, I will pass over you; and the plague shall not be on you to destroy you when I strike the land of Egypt."

Revelation 12:11

"And they overcame him by the blood of the Lamb and by the word of their testimony, and they did not love their lives to the death."

CHAPTER 3

*GOD WANTS ALL HIS CHILDREN
HEALED AND IN HEALTH*

Luke 13:10-18

10 "Now He was teaching in one of the synagogues on the Sabbath.

11 And behold, there was a woman who had a spirit of infirmity eighteen years, and was bent over and could in no way raise herself up.

12 But when Jesus saw her, He called her to Him and said to her, "Woman, you are loosed from your infirmity."

13 And He laid His hands on her, and immediately she was made straight, and glorified God.

14 But the ruler of the synagogue answered with indignation, because Jesus had healed on the Sabbath; and he said to the crowd, "There are six days on which men ought to work; therefore, come and be healed on them, and not on the Sabbath day."

15 The Lord then answered him and said, "Hypocrite! Does not each one of you on the Sabbath lose his ox or donkey from the stall, and lead it away to water it?

16 "So ought not this woman, being a daughter of Abraham, whom Satan has bound--think of it--for eighteen years, be loosed from this bond on the Sabbath?"

17 And when He said these things, all His adversaries were put to shame; and all the multitude rejoiced for all the glorious things that were done by Him.

18 Then He said, "What is the kingdom of God like? And to what shall I compare it?"

Abraham's Daughter was healed.

Galatians 3:29

"And if you are Christ's, then you are Abraham's seed, and heirs according to the promise."

If you be born again (Christ's, then are ye Abraham's seed and heirs (of God) according to the promise.

If Jesus wanted Abraham's daughter made whole (in Luke 13:10-18) then Hebrews 13:8 shows He equally wants you made whole today. It's up to you.

Exodus 15:26

And if you are Christ's, then you are Abraham's seed, and heirs according to the promise.

Exodus 23:25-26

25 "So you shall serve the LORD your God, and He will bless your bread and your water. And I will take sickness away from the midst of you.

26 "No one shall suffer miscarriage or be barren in your land; I will fulfill the number of your days."

Deuteronomy 7:11-15

11 "Therefore you shall keep the commandment, the statutes, and the judgments which I command you today, to observe them.

12 "Then it shall come to pass, because you listen to these judgments, and keep and do them, that the LORD your God will keep with you the covenant and the mercy which He swore to your fathers.

13 "And He will love you and bless you and multiply you; He will also bless the fruit of your womb and the fruit of your land, your grain and your new wine and your oil, the increase of your cattle and the offspring of your flock, in the land of which He swore to your fathers to give you.

14 "You shall be blessed above all peoples; there shall not be a

male or female barren among you or among your livestock.

15 "And the LORD will take away from you all sickness, and will afflict you with none of the terrible diseases of Egypt which you have known, but will lay them on all those who hate you."

Malachi 3:6

"For I am the LORD, I do not change; Therefore, you are not consumed, O sons of Jacob."

Hebrews 13:8

"Jesus Christ is the same yesterday, today, and forever."

Psalms 82:6

I said, "You are gods, and all of you are children of the Most High."

John 10:34-35

34 Jesus answered them, "Is it not written in your law, 'I said, "You are gods"'?

35 "If He called them gods, to whom the word of God came (and the Scripture cannot be broken),"

Romans 8:14-16

14 "For as many as are led by the Spirit of God, these are sons of God.

15 For you did not receive the spirit of bondage again to fear, but you received the Spirit of adoption by whom we cry out, "Abba, Father."

16 The Spirit Himself bears witness with our spirit that we are children of God,"

Galatians 4:6-7

6 "And because you are sons, God has sent forth the Spirit of His Son into your hearts, crying out, "Abba, Father!"

7 Therefore you are no longer a slave but a son, and if a son, then an heir of God through Christ."

Therefore, we are not to be sick just as Jesus was never sick.

SOURCES OF SICKNESS/DISEASE.

1. Satan

Acts 10:38

"how God anointed Jesus of Nazareth with the Holy Spirit and with power, who went about doing good and healing all who were oppressed by the devil, for God was with Him."

Luke 13:10-17

10 "Now He was teaching in one of the synagogues on the Sabbath.

11 And behold, there was a woman who had a spirit of infirmity eighteen years, and was bent over and could in no way raise herself up.

12 But when Jesus saw her, He called her to Him and said to her, "Woman, you are loosed from your infirmity."

13 And He laid His hands on her, and immediately she was made straight, and glorified God.

14 But the ruler of the synagogue answered with indignation, because Jesus had healed on the Sabbath; and he said to the crowd, "There are six days on which men ought to work; therefore, come and be healed on them, and not on the Sabbath day."

15 The Lord then answered him and said, "Hypocrite! Does not each one of you on the Sabbath lose his ox or donkey from the stall, and lead it away to water it?

16 "So ought not this woman, being a daughter of Abraham, whom Satan has bound--think of it--for eighteen years, be loosed from this bond on the Sabbath?"

17 And when He said these things, all His adversaries were put to shame; and all the multitude rejoiced for all the glorious things that were done by Him."

James 5:7

"Therefore, be patient, brethren, until the coming of the Lord. See how the farmer waits for the precious fruit of the earth, waiting patiently for it until it receives the early and latter rain."

1 Peter 5:9

"Resist him, steadfast in the faith, knowing that the same sufferings are experienced by your brotherhood in the world."

John 10:10

"The thief does not come except to steal, and to kill, and to destroy. I have come that they may have life, and that they may have it more abundantly."

2. Wrong Confession.

Proverbs 18:20-21

20 "A man's stomach shall be satisfied from the fruit of his mouth; From the produce of his lips he shall be filled.

21 Death and life are in the power of the tongue, and those who love it will eat its fruit."

James 3:1-9

1 "My brethren, let not many of you become teachers, knowing that we shall receive a stricter judgment.

2 For we all stumble in many things. If anyone does not stumble in word, he is a perfect man, able also to bridle the whole body.

3 Indeed, we put bits in horses' mouths that they may obey us, and we turn their whole body.

4 Look also at ships: although they are so large and are driven by fierce winds, they are turned by a very small rudder wherever the pilot desires.

5 Even so the tongue is a little member and boasts great things. See how great a forest a little fire kindles!

6 And the tongue is a fire, a world of iniquity. The tongue is so set among our members that it defiles the whole body, and sets on fire the course of nature; and it is set on fire by hell.

7 For every kind of beast and bird, of reptile and creature of the sea, is tamed and has been tamed by mankind.

8 But no man can tame the tongue. It is an unruly evil, full of deadly poison.

9 With it we bless our God and Father, and with it we curse men, who have been made in the similitude of God."

Job 1:5

"So it was, when the days of feasting had run their course, that Job would send and sanctify them, and he would rise early in the morning and offer burnt offerings according to the number of them all. For Job said, "It may be that my sons have sinned and cursed God in their hearts." Thus, Job did regularly."

Proverbs 6:2

"You are snared by the words of your mouth; You are taken by the words of your mouth."

3. Wrong Thinking.

Proverbs 23:7

"For as he thinks in his heart, so is he. "Eat and drink!" he says to you, but his heart is not with you."

4. Selfishness, stinginess and withholding back from giving.

James 5:1-4

"Therefore, be patient, brethren, until the coming of the Lord. See how the farmer waits for the precious fruit of the earth, waiting patiently for it until it receives the early and latter rain."

1 Timithy 6:10-12

10 "For the love of money is a root of all kinds of evil, for which some have strayed from the faith in their greediness, and pierced themselves through with many sorrows.

11 But you, O man of God, flee these things and pursue righteousness, godliness, faith, love, patience, gentleness.

12 Fight the good fight of faith, lay hold on eternal life, to which you were also called and have confessed the good confession in the presence of many witnesses."

Job 4:2-10

2 "If one attempts a word with you, will you become weary? But who can withhold himself from speaking?

3 Surely you have instructed many, and you have strengthened weak hands.

4 Your words have upheld him who was stumbling, and you have strengthened the feeble knees;

5 But now it comes upon you, and you are weary; It touches you, and you are troubled.

6 Is not your reverence your confidence? And the integrity of your ways your hope?

7 "Remember now, whoever perished being innocent? Or where were the upright ever cut off?

8 Even as I have seen, those who plow iniquity and sow trouble reap the same.

9 By the blast of God they perish, and by the breath of His anger they are consumed.

10 The roaring of the lion, the voice of the fierce lion, And the teeth of the young lions are broken."

5. Disobedience to The Living Word.

Deuteronomy 28:15-68

15 "But it shall come to pass, if you do not obey the voice of the LORD your God, to observe carefully all His commandments and His statutes which I command you today, that all these curses will come upon you and overtake you:

16 "Cursed shall you be in the city, and cursed shall you be in the country.

17 "Cursed shall be your basket and your kneading bowl.

18 "Cursed shall be the fruit of your body and the produce of your land, the increase of your cattle and the offspring of your flocks.

19 "Cursed shall you be when you come in, and cursed shall you be when you go out.

20 "The LORD will send on you cursing, confusion, and rebuke in all that you set your hand to do, until you are destroyed and until you perish quickly, because of the wickedness of your doings in which you have forsaken Me.

21 "The LORD will make the plague cling to you until He has consumed you from the land which you are going to possess.

22 "The LORD will strike you with consumption, with fever, with inflammation, with severe burning fever, with the sword, with scorching, and with mildew; they shall pursue you until you perish.

23 "And your heavens which are over your head shall be bronze, and the earth which is under you shall be iron.

24 "The LORD will change the rain of your land to powder and dust; from the heaven it shall come down on you until you are destroyed.

25 "The LORD will cause you to be defeated before your enemies; you shall go out one way against them and flee seven ways before them; and you shall become troublesome to all the kingdoms of the earth.

26 "Your carcasses shall be food for all the birds of the air and the beasts of the earth, and no one shall frighten them away.

27 "The LORD will strike you with the boils of Egypt, with tu-

mors, with the scab, and with the itch, from which you cannot be healed.

28 "The LORD will strike you with madness and blindness and confusion of heart.

29 "And you shall grope at noonday, as a blind man gropes in darkness; you shall not prosper in your ways; you shall be only oppressed and plundered continually, and no one shall save you.

30 "You shall betroth a wife, but another man shall lie with her; you shall build a house, but you shall not dwell in it; you shall plant a vineyard, but shall not gather its grapes.

31 "Your ox shall be slaughtered before your eyes, but you shall not eat of it; your donkey shall be violently taken away from before you, and shall not be restored to you; your sheep shall be given to your enemies, and you shall have no one to rescue them.

32 "Your sons and your daughters shall be given to another people, and your eyes shall look and fail with longing for them all day long; and there shall be no strength in your hand.

33 "A nation whom you have not known shall eat the fruit of your land and the produce of your labor, and you shall be only oppressed and crushed continually.

34 "So you shall be driven mad because of the sight which your eyes see.

35 "The LORD will strike you in the knees and on the legs with severe boils which cannot be healed, and from the sole of your foot to the top of your head.

36 "The LORD will bring you and the king whom you set over you to a nation which neither you nor your fathers have known, and there you shall serve other gods-wood and stone.

37 "And you shall become an astonishment, a proverb, and a byword among all nations where the LORD will drive you.

38 "You shall carry much seed out to the field but gather little in, for the locust shall consume it.

39 "You shall plant vineyards and tend them, but you shall neither drink of the wine nor gather the grapes; for the worms shall eat them.

40 "You shall have olive trees throughout all your territory, but

you shall not anoint yourself with the oil; for your olives shall drop off.

41 "You shall beget sons and daughters, but they shall not be yours; for they shall go into captivity.

42 "Locusts shall consume all your trees and the produce of your land.

43 "The alien who is among you shall rise higher and higher above you, and you shall come down lower and lower.

44 "He shall lend to you, but you shall not lend to him; he shall be the head, and you shall be the tail.

45 "Moreover all these curses shall come upon you and pursue and overtake you, until you are destroyed, because you did not obey the voice of the LORD your God, to keep His commandments and His statutes which He commanded you.

46 "And they shall be upon you for a sign and a wonder, and on your descendants forever.

47 "Because you did not serve the LORD your God with joy and gladness of heart, for the abundance of everything,

48 "therefore you shall serve your enemies, whom the LORD will send against you, in hunger, in thirst, in nakedness, and in need of everything; and He will put a yoke of iron on your neck until He has destroyed you.

49 "The LORD will bring a nation against you from afar, from the end of the earth, as swift as the eagle flies, a nation whose language you will not understand,

50 "a nation of fierce countenance, which does not respect the elderly nor show favor to the young.

51 "And they shall eat the increase of your livestock and the produce of your land, until you are destroyed; they shall not leave you grain or new wine or oil, or the increase of your cattle or the offspring of your flocks, until they have destroyed you.

52 "They shall besiege you at all your gates until your high and fortified walls, in which you trust, come down throughout all your land; and they shall besiege you at all your gates throughout all your land which the LORD your God has given you.

53 "You shall eat the fruit of your own body, the flesh of your

sons and your daughters whom the LORD your God has given you, in the siege and desperate straits in which your enemy shall distress you.

54 "The sensitive and very refined man among you will be hostile toward his brother, toward the wife of his bosom, and toward the rest of his children whom he leaves behind,

55 "so that he will not give any of them the flesh of his children whom he will eat, because he has nothing left in the siege and desperate straits in which your enemy shall distress you at all your gates.

56 "The tender and delicate woman among you, who would not venture to set the sole of her foot on the ground because of her delicateness and sensitivity, will refuse to the husband of her bosom, and to her son and her daughter,

57 "her placenta which comes out from between her feet and her children whom she bears; for she will eat them secretly for lack of everything in the siege and desperate straits in which your enemy shall distress you at all your gates.

58 "If you do not carefully observe all the words of this law that are written in this book, that you may fear this glorious and awesome name, THE LORD YOUR GOD,

59 "then the LORD will bring upon you and your descendants extraordinary plagues-great and prolonged plagues-and serious and prolonged sicknesses.

60 "Moreover He will bring back on you all the diseases of Egypt, of which you were afraid, and they shall cling to you.

61 "Also every sickness and every plague, which is not written in this Book of the Law, will the LORD bring upon you until you are destroyed.

62 "You shall be left few in number, whereas you were as the stars of heaven in multitude, because you would not obey the voice of the LORD your God.

63 "And it shall be, that just as the LORD rejoiced over you to do you good and multiply you, so the LORD will rejoice over you to destroy you and bring you to nothing; and you shall be plucked from off the land which you go to possess.

64 "Then the LORD will scatter you among all peoples, from one end of the earth to the other, and there you shall serve other gods, which neither you nor your fathers have known-wood and stone.

65 "And among those nations you shall find no rest, nor shall the sole of your foot have a resting place; but there the L ORD will give you a trembling heart, failing eyes, and anguish of soul.

66 "Your life shall hang in doubt before you; you shall fear day and night, and have no assurance of life.

67 "In the morning you shall say, 'Oh, that it was evening!' And at evening you shall say, 'Oh, that it was morning!' because of the fear which terrifies your heart, and because of the sight which your eyes see.

68 "And the LORD will take you back to Egypt in ships, by the way of which I said to you, 'You shall never see it again.' And there you shall be offered for sale to your enemies as male and female slaves, but no one will buy you."

6. Not serving with joy/gladness.

Psalms 100:2

"Serve the LORD with gladness; Come before His presence with singing."

Deuteronomy 28:47-48

47 "Because you did not serve the LORD your God with joy and gladness of heart, for the abundance of everything,

48 "therefore you shall serve your enemies, whom the LORD will send against you, in hunger, in thirst, in nakedness, and in need of everything; and He will put a yoke of iron on your neck until He has destroyed you."

7. Fear.

Job 3:25

"For the thing I greatly feared has come upon me, and what I dreaded has happened to me."

8. Ignorance/lack of knowledge.

Hosea 4:6

"My people are destroyed for lack of knowledge. Because you have rejected knowledge, I also will reject you from being priest for Me; Because you have forgotten the law of your God, I also will forget your children."

Isaiah 5:13

"Therefore, my people have gone into captivity, because they have no knowledge; Their honorable men are famished, and their multitude dried up with thirst."

Psalms 82:5-7

5 "They do not know, nor do they understand; They walk about in darkness; All the foundations of the earth are unstable.

6 I said, "You are gods, and all of you are children of the Most High.

7 But you shall die like men, and fall like one of the princes."

9. The curse, Deuteronomy 28:15-68.

Galatians 2:16-17

15 "We who are Jews by nature, and not sinners of the Gentiles,

16 "knowing that a man is not justified by the works of the law but by faith in Jesus Christ, even we have believed in Christ Jesus, that we might be justified by faith in Christ and not by the works of the law; for by the works of the law no flesh shall be justified.

17 "But if, while we seek to be justified by Christ, we ourselves also are found sinners, is Christ therefore a minister of sin? Certainly not!"

10. Sin.

Romans 3:23

"for all have sinned and fall short of the glory of God,"

Romans 6:23

"For all have sinned and fall short of the glory of God,"

Genesis 2:16-17

16 "And the LORD God commanded the man, saying, "Of every tree of the garden you may freely eat;

17 "but of the tree of the knowledge of good and evil you shall not eat, for in the day that you eat of it you shall surely die."

11. Over-work (Epaphroditus)

Philippians 2:25-27

25 "Yet I considered it necessary to send to you Epaphroditus, my brother, fellow worker, and fellow soldier, but your messen-

ger and the one who ministered to my need;

26 since he was longing for you all, and was distressed because you had heard that he was sick.

27 For indeed he was sick almost unto death; but God had mercy on him, and not only on him but on me also, lest I should have sorrow upon sorrow."

Ecclesiastes 10:15

"The labor of fools wearies them, for they do not even know how to go to the city!"

12. Breaking the Covenant.

"But it shall come to pass, if you do not obey the voice of the LORD your God, to observe carefully all His commandments and His statutes which I command you today, that all these curses will come upon you and overtake you: "If you do not carefully observe all the words of this law that are written in this book, that you may fear this glorious and awesome name, THE LORD YOUR GOD, "then the LORD will bring upon you and your descendants extraordinary plagues-great and prolonged plagues-and serious and prolonged sicknesses. Moreover, He will bring back on you all the diseases of Egypt, of which you were afraid, and they shall cling to you. Also, every sickness and every plague, which is not written in this Book of the Law, will the LORD bring upon you until you are destroyed." Deuteronomy 28:15,58-61

13. Not working in love.

1John 3:14

"We know that we have passed from death to life, because we love the brethren. He who does not love his brother abides in death."

14. Hatred of God's covenant/obedient heirs.

Deuteronomy 7:15

"And the LORD will take away from you all sickness, and will afflict you with none of the terrible diseases of Egypt which you have known, but will lay them on all those who hate you."

15. Bringing an abominable/devoted thing into your house.

Deuteronomy 7:26

"Nor shall you bring an abomination into your house, lest you be doomed to destruction like it. You shall utterly detest it and utterly abhor it, for it is an accursed thing."

Malachi 3:8-9

8 "Will a man rob God? Yet you have robbed Me! But you say, 'In what way have we robbed You?' In tithes and offerings.

9 You are cursed with a curse, for you have robbed Me, Even this whole nation."

Zechariah 5:1-4

1 "Then I turned and raised my eyes, and saw there a flying scroll.

2 And he said to me, "What do you see?" So, I answered, "I see a flying scroll. Its length is twenty cubits and its width ten cubits."

3 Then he said to me, "This is the curse that goes out over the face of the whole earth: 'Every thief shall be expelled,' according to this side of the scroll; and, 'Every perjurer shall be expelled,' according to that side of it."

4 "I will send out the curse," says the LORD of hosts; "It shall enter the house of the thief and the house of the one who swears falsely by My name. It shall remain in the midst of his house and consume it, with its timber and stones."

Joshua 7:10-13

10 "So the LORD said to Joshua: "Get up! Why do you lie thus on your face?

11 "Israel has sinned, and they have also transgressed My covenant which I commanded them. For they have even taken some of the accursed things, and have both stolen and deceived; and they have also put it among their own stuff.

12 "Therefore the children of Israel could not stand before their enemies, but turned their backs before their enemies, because they have become doomed to destruction. Neither will I be with you anymore, unless you destroy the accursed from among you.

13 "Get up, sanctify the people, and say, 'Sanctify yourselves for tomorrow, because thus says the LORD God of Israel: "There is an accursed thing in your midst, O Israel; you cannot stand before your enemies until you take away the accursed thing from among you."

CHAPTER 4

THE REASON FOR THE CHURCH IS FOR ALL TO BE HEALED

THE REASON FOR THE CHURCH IS FOR ALL TO BE HEALED! AND THE LORD'S PRESENCE AND HIS POWER ARE ALWAYS AVAILABLE TO HEAL HIS PEOPLE WHEN WE ARE GATHERED TOGETHER!

Hebrews 10:25

"Not forsaking the assembling of ourselves together, as is the manner of some, but exhorting one another, and so much the more as you see the Day approaching."

(NIV) Let us not give up meeting together, as some are in the habit of doing...

Please Note:

1Corinthians 5:4

"In the name of our Lord Jesus Christ, when you are gathered together, along with my spirit, with the power of our Lord Jesus Christ,"

Luke 5:17

"Now it happened on a certain day, as He was teaching, that there were Pharisees and teachers of the law sitting by, who had come out of every town of Galilee, Judea, and Jerusalem. And the power of the Lord was present to heal them."

Psalms 133:1-3 (NIV)

1 "How good and pleasant it is when brothers live(dwell) together in unity!

2 it is like precious oil poured on the head, running down on the beard, running down on Aaron's beard, down upon the collar of his robes.

3 it is as if the dew of Hermon were falling on mount Zion. For there the Lord bestows his blessings, even life forever more.

Matthew 18:16,18-20 (NIV)

16 "But if he will not listen, take one or two others along (making 2 or 3 of you), so that "EVERY MATTER MAY BE ESTABLISHED BY THE TESTIMONY OF TWO OR THREE WITNESSES.

18 I tell you the truth, whatever you bind on earth will be bound in heaven, and whatever you lose on earth will be loosed in heaven.

19 Again, I tell you (Emphatically) that if two of you on earth agree about anything you ask for, it will be done for you by my Father in heaven.

20. For where two or three come together in my name, there am I with them."

1 Corinthians 5:4

When you are assembled in the name of our Lord Jesus and I am with you in spirit, and the POWER OF OUR LORD JESUS IS PRESENT.

Note: Paul says "I am with you in spirit" when you are assembled in the Name of our Lord Jesus.

Hebrews 12:22-24 shows that the spirit of just men made perfect is present whenever/wherever the people of God are assembled together.

It is also clearly shown that THE POWER OF OUR LORD JESUS IS PRESENT. For what purpose?

Luke 5:17 (NIV)

"...and the POWER OF THE LORD was present for Him to heal the sick."

Where 2 or 3 are gathered together, the LORD is there.

Wherever the LORD is present, there His power is PRESENT.

And wherever the power of the LORD is present, the purpose of the LORD'S power present is to HEAL THE SICK.

Therefore, no trace of sickness will be found in you anymore.

Acts 10:38 (NIV)

How God anointed Jesus of Nazareth with the Holy Spirit and power, and how he went around doing good and HEALING ALL WHO were under the power of the devil, because God was with him.

That is why I know beyond and far above all doubts that there is no day we shall gather anywhere as believers (His church) in His Name that the LORD will not be present in His fullness of power to Heal all the sick who are under the devil's power and oppression.

Our gathering together in His Name is enough to terminate all sickness/disease even without our praying and asking Him to Heal the sick.

Our gathering together in the Name of the Lord Jesus commands His presence and power and the release of His Blessings-Healing, Health, Prosperity, abundances, salvation, life-all the blessings of the Lord.

This is why those who have anyone sick should endeavor to ensure they bring their sick ones to church instead of pushing them to the hospital-even if it means living a hearse.

See Matthew 8:16

"When evening had come, they brought to Him many who were demon-possessed. And He cast out the spirits with a word, and healed all who were sick,"

Matthew 4:24

"Then His fame went throughout all Syria; and they brought to Him all sick people who were afflicted with various diseases and torments, and those who were demon-possessed, epileptics, and paralytics; and He healed them."

Matthew 12:15

"But when Jesus knew it, He withdrew from there. And great multitudes followed Him, and He healed them all."

Matthew 14:13-14,34-36

13 "When Jesus heard it, He departed from there by boat to a deserted place by Himself. But when the multitudes heard it, they followed Him on foot from the cities.

14 And when Jesus went out, He saw a great multitude; and He was moved with compassion for them, and healed their sick.

34 When they had crossed over, they came to the land of Gennesaret.

35 And when the men of that place recognized Him, they sent out into all that surrounding region, brought to Him all who were sick,

36 and begged Him that they might only touch the hem of His garment. And as many as touched it were made perfectly well."

Matthew 15:30-31

30 "Then great multitudes came to Him, having with them the lame, blind, mute, maimed, and many others; and they laid them down at Jesus' feet, and He healed them.

31 So the multitude marveled when they saw the mute speaking, the maimed made whole, the lame walking, and the blind seeing; and they glorified the God of Israel."

Mathew 21:14

"Then the blind and the lame came to Him in the temple, and He healed them."

Mark 1:32-34

32 "At evening, when the sun had set, they brought to Him all who were sick and those who were demon-possessed.

33 And the whole city was gathered together at the door.

34 Then He healed many who were sick with various diseases, and cast out many demons; and He did not allow the demons to speak, because they knew Him."

Mark 3:7-10

7 "But Jesus withdrew with His disciples to the sea. And a great multitude from Galilee followed Him, and from Judea

8 and Jerusalem and Idumea and beyond the Jordan; and those from Tyre and Sidon, a great multitude, when they heard how many things He was doing, came to Him.

9 So He told His disciples that a small boat should be kept ready

for Him because of the multitude, lest they should crush Him.

10 For He healed many, so that as many as had afflictions pressed about Him to touch Him."

Luke 4:40

"When the sun was setting, all those who had any that were sick with various diseases brought them to Him; and He laid His hands on every one of them and healed them."

Luke 5:17

"Now it happened on a certain day, as He was teaching, that there were Pharisees and teachers of the law sitting by, who had come out of every town of Galilee, Judea, and Jerusalem. And the power of the Lord was present to heal them."

Luke 6:17-19

17 "And He came down with them and stood on a level place with a crowd of His disciples and a great multitude of people from all Judea and Jerusalem, and from the seacoast of Tyre and Sidon, who came to hear Him and be healed of their diseases,

18 as well as those who were tormented with unclean spirits. And they were healed.

19 And the whole multitude sought to touch Him, for power went out from Him and healed them all."

Acts 2:42-44

42 "And they continued steadfastly in the apostles' doctrine and fellowship, in the breaking of bread, and in prayers.

43 Then fear came upon every soul, and many wonders and signs were done through the apostles.

44 Now all who believed were together, and had all things in common,"

Acts 5:12-16

12 "And through the hands of the apostles many signs and wonders were done among the people. And they were all with one accord in Solomon's Porch.

13 Yet none of the rest dared join them, but the people esteemed them highly.

14 And believers were increasingly added to the Lord, multitudes of both men and women,

15 so that they brought the sick out into the streets and laid them on beds and couches, that at least the shadow of Peter passing by might fall on some of them.

16 Also a multitude gathered from the surrounding cities to Jerusalem, bringing sick people and those who were tormented by unclean spirits, and they were all healed."

Acts 28:8-9

8 "And it happened that the father of Publius lay sick of a fever and dysentery. Paul went in to him and prayed, and he laid his hands on him and healed him.

9 So when this was done, the rest of those on the island who had diseases also came and were healed."

The power of the LORD is always present wherever His own people gather together in His Name. And the reason for the presence of His power is to HEAL THE SICK. Luke 5:17; Matthew 18:20

The ignorance of the church to this truth has kept so many in bondage to sickness/disease and under the power of the devil-Isaiah 5:13; Hosea 4:6; Psalms 82:5-7.

John 8:31-32,36-knowledge/understanding of the truth is what makes for freedom. From now, none Calmers who worship here and dwells in our midst in unity with the saints of God will ever be sick.

I decree henceforth you shall enjoy the health or healing or blessings His presence and His power bestows on His people. So, shall it be in Jesus Name.

Warning.

Proverbs 16:28B

"And a whisperer separates the best of friends."

Beware you don't walk in disunity.

Proverbs 16:28B

"And a whisperer separates the best of friends."

Make sure you are not divisive.

Beware you don't sow discord among brethren.

Proverbs 16:28A

"A perverse man sows strife."

Beware you don't walk in strife.

Proverbs 16:30B

"He purses his lips and brings about evil."

Beware you are not a talebearer.

Proverbs 19:17

"He who has pity on the poor lends to the LORD, And He will pay back what he has given."

Beware your words don't cause others to err.

Proverbs 6:2A

"You are snared by the words of your mouth;"

Beware you don't speak evil words.

Proverbs 18:20-21

20 "A man's stomach shall be satisfied from the fruit of his mouth; From the produce of his lips he shall be filled.

21 Death and life are in the power of the tongue, and those who love it will eat its fruit."

Beware you don't speak curses/death.

Proverbs 18:7

"A fool's mouth is his destruction, and his lips are the snare of his soul."

Beware you don't speak like a fool-(Psalms 14:1ff, 53:1ff).

Remember Psalms 107:20; Psalms 68:11 and Proverbs 13:17.

The Lord sent his word and healed them and delivered then from their destructions.

The Lord sent the word and great was the company of those who published it.

We are only here to publish the word He sent and healed them and delivered them from their destructions. We are Calmers-Ambassadors of health-sent here as Jesus was sent to bring good and healing to all. (Psalms 107:20; Acts 10:38; Proverbs 13:17; John 14:12; John 17:18; John 20:21; Psalms 68:11).

We must maintain fellowship (Acts 2:42-44; 4:32-35; Acts 5:12-16). And we must learn to speak only the words of life that we have been given.

Remember the Lord is Present where Calmers are. And His power is present to Heal the sick.

No sick person must come into our midst for fellowship and leave/return sick. This knowledge will enforce their healing in Jesus Name.

Jeremiah 1:12

Then the LORD said to me, "You have seen well, for I am ready to perform My word."

Psalms 89:34

"My covenant I will not break, nor alter the word that has gone out of My lips."

Isaiah 45:23

"I have sworn by Myself; The word has gone out of My mouth in righteousness, and shall not return, That to Me every knee shall bow, every tongue shall take an oath."

Isaiah 55:8-11

8 "For My thoughts are not your thoughts, nor are your ways My ways," says the LORD.

9 "For as the heavens are higher than the earth, so are My ways higher than your ways, And My thoughts than your thoughts.

10 "For as the rain comes down, and the snow from heaven, and do not return there, but water the earth, and make it bring forth and bud, that it may give seed to the sower and bread to the eater,

11 So shall My word be that goes forth from My mouth; It shall not return to Me void, but it shall accomplish what I please, and it shall prosper in the thing for which I sent it."

Psalms 119:89

"Forever, O LORD, your word is settled in heaven."

Please Note:

1Corinthians 6:14 (NIV)

By his power God Raised the LORD from the dead, AND HE WILL RAISE US ALSO (BY HIS POWER).

Romans 1:4 (NIV) (1Corinthians 6:19-20; Ephesians 3:20).

His power is present to Raise the dead in our midst. 1Corinthians 15:42-44.

And who through the Spirit of his likeness was declared with POWER to be the son of God, by his resurrection from the dead. Jesus Christ our Lord. (See Acts 2:240). The presence of his power destroys the power of sin, pain, sickness and death. Luke 10:19; Hebrews 2:14-15.

Romans 8:11 (NIV)

And if the Spirit of him who raised Jesus from the dead is living in you, he who raised Christ from the dead will also give life to your mortal bodies through his Spirit, who lives in you.

1Corinthians 5:4; Luke 5:17(NIV)...the power of the Lord is present ...and the power of the Lord is present to heal the sick.

CHAPTER 5

J esus never imposed conditions before healing man from sin and sickness and disease once He sees faith in such person.

The law is overruled by faith and on the basis of faith the Lord performs miracles of healing and deliverance.

Faith is the ultimate. Raise/Build/Increase their faith, then impossible cases will be healed and made possible.

If Faith was there, that was all Jesus wanted. Show All the way of Faith. It is the pathway to their victory over all.

Psalms 107:20

All of creation's sickness springs from within. The Living Word must be sent to Heal All.

Politics, Industry, Banking, Organizations, Agriculture, Medicine, Education, Mankind, Animals, Companies, Lands, Nations, States, Departments, Faculties, etc need healing. So, Heal all.

So, Healing begins from within. Heal the inside (within) and outside will be healed.

CHAPTER 6

GOD'S ORDER OF PRIORITY

1.Give The Living Word to All.

2.Heal Them.

3.Deliver Them.

Psalms 107:20 (RSV)

"He sent forth his word, and healed them, and delivered them from destruction." "Them" talks about the Israel of God, not mankind or the world.

Deuteronomy 34:7

"Moses was one hundred and twenty years old when he died. His eyes were not dim nor his natural vigor diminished."

Hebrew 8:7

"For if that first covenant had been faultless, then no place would have been sought for a second."

Psalms 68:11 (KJV)

"The Lord gave the word: great was the company of those that published it."

1. The Lord sent forth his word or gave the word (first).

The word the Lord sent forth was/is given to the world (mankind) by those he sent (Romans 10:13-15; Psalms 68:11).

They taught/preached the message/word they were given and sent to preach (See also Isaiah 44:26).

Luke 5:17

And it came to pass on a certain day, as he was teaching, that there were Pharisees and doctors of the law sitting by, which were come out of every town of Galilee, and Judaea, and Jerusalem: and the power of the Lord was present to heal them.

Jesus taught The Living Word.

Luke 18-Jesus preached The Living Word

Mark 4:23; 9:35-Jesus taught/preached The Living Word.

Therefore, the first thing in God's priority is give the world or mankind- the poor, the sick, the bound, the afflicted, the captives, the blind, the brokenhearted, the sinners, the unbelievers, all of mankind- The Living Word. Give all the word first. This is God's topmost priority in His order of events. The Living Word is first. Give The Living Word first to all no matter their situations.

John 1:1-5

1 "In the beginning was the Word, and the Word was with God, and the Word was God.

2 The same was in the beginning with God.

3 All things were made by him; and without him was not anything made that was made.

4 In him was life; and the life was the light of men.

5 And the light shineth in darkness; and the darkness comprehended it not." The Living word is God and God is first and last.

Don't place anything above The Living Word in priority. The Living Word must be first/the beginning. Let The Living Word here preeminence over all. Teach, Preach, give, and send forth The Living Word first.

2. After giving The Living Word, then Heal All the sick.

The Lord sent forth or gave The Living Word AND HEALED THEM.

God didn't make altar call for souls to be saved after giving the Living Word. He taught/preached/gave/sent forth The Living Word and afterwards HE HEALED THEM that were sick.

This clearly shows that God is very practical about the redemption of man. He healed them after He gave them The Living Word. Therefore, after teaching/preaching/giving/sending forth The Living Word, heal them that had need of healing. This is second in God's order of priority-Healing is second, - after Teaching/preaching.

Matthew 4:23

"And Jesus went about all Galilee, teaching in their synagogues, and preaching the gospel of the kingdom, and healing all manner of sickness and all manner of disease among the people."

Matthew 9:35

"And Jesus went about all the cities and villages, teaching in their synagogues, and preaching the gospel of the kingdom, and healing every sickness and every disease among the people."

Teaching/preaching/giving The Living Word, then HEALING.

3. After teaching them The Living Word and Healing them, then the 3rd thing in God's order of priority is Deliverance/salvation.

He sent forth (gave) His word and Healed them and delivered them from their destructions.

Deliverance from their destructions covers salvation from sin, salvation from poverty, salvation from bondage/captivity/enslavement. Deliverance from their destructions covers emancipation from whatever is after man's destructions (Luke 4:18-19; Romans 8:19-22). This clearly shows that deliverance from sin and all forms of bondages/enslavements/afflictions is 3RD in God's priority after Giving The Living Word and Healing them.

1.Teach/Preach/Send forth/Give them The Living Word first.

2.Heal them that has need of healing is second.

3.Deliver them from whatever is after their destructions is third in God's order of priority.

Most of the time, preachers preach The Living Word and make alter call for sinners to be delivered. This is all they do. Evangelists also do the same.

Pastors equally preach the Living Word and at times make alter calls or at times don't depending on the time they have.

Teachers teach The Living Word and may or may not make alter calls.

Apostles, Prophets, Bishops, etc Teach/preach and may or may not make alter calls depending on the moods and that of their congregation. They are all falters as they have failed to carry out God's purpose. Their neglect of God's priority is the reason for the state of the church and the suffering of the world (mankind).

God's priority is Teach/Preach The Living Word, then Heal, then Save or deliver, or liberate, or emancipate them that are suffering in Satanic enslavements no matter what their problems may be. (Luke 4:18-19; Matthew 25:31-40; Isaiah 58:6-8).

Every messenger sent by God is to-

-Teach/Preach The Living Word First.

- Heal the sick secondly, and

- Deliver them from their destructions, thirdly.

To fail to do any of the above or to jump any or to ignore any because of any reason is to fail to do what you have been sent to do.

Psalm 68:11

"The Lord gave the word: great was the company of those that published it."

Psalms 107:20

"He sent his word, and healed them, and delivered them from their destructions."

Isaiah 44:26

"That confirms the word of his servant, and performeth the counsel of his messengers; that says to Jerusalem, thou shalt be inhabited; and to the cities of Judah, Ye shall be built, and I will raise up the decayed places thereof:"

Mark 16:19-20

19 "So then after the Lord had spoken unto them, he was received up into heaven, and sat on the right hand of God.

20 And they went forth, and preached everywhere, the Lord working with them, and confirming the word with signs following. Amen."

The above scriptures show very clearly that when we do it the way He has commanded it, He confirms The Living Word by doing as He says.

But we must follow His order of priority.

Most preachers see dying humanity and preach The Living Word and make or refuse to make alter calls and stroll away believing they have done their best.

Psalms 107:20- God gave The Living Word first.

God Healed them secondly.

God delivered them from their destructions thirdly.

Matthew 4:23, 9:35- Jesus Taught/preached The Living Word first (Luke 4:18A.

Jesus healed All the sick second. (Matthew 4:23; 9:35).

Jesus delivered them from their destructions. (Luke 418-19,40-44).

He did so because God was with Him (Acts 10:38, 2:22).

There was nothing Jesus ever did on his own. The father was the one who did all this works through Jesus (John 5:17-19, etc).

John 17:18; 20:21; 14:12- We are here to do not our own works the way we want it but the same works the father sent Him to do As He did it. We are to follow His first steps. (1Peter 2:21).

God/Jesus gave The Living Word first.

God/Jesus Healed them secondly.

God/Jesus Delivered them from their destructions.

We must Do likewise.

WHAT ARE THEIR DESTRUCTIONS?

1.Ignorance

Hosea 4:6

"My people are destroyed for lack of knowledge: because thou hast rejected knowledge, I will also reject thee, that thou shalt be no priest to me: seeing thou hast forgotten the law of thy God, I will also forget thy children."

Isaiah 5:13

"Therefore, my people are gone into captivity, because they have no knowledge: and their honourable men are famished, and their multitude dried up with thirst."

Psalms 82:5-7

5 "They know not, neither will they understand; they walk on in darkness: all the foundations of the earth are out of course.

6 I have said, Ye are gods; and all of you are children of the most High.

7 But ye shall die like men, and fall like one of the princes."

2. Poverty

Proverbs 10:15

"The rich man's wealth is his strong city: the destruction of the poor is their poverty." (Proverbs 13:8)

3. Unbelief/Sin

Romans 14:23

"And he that doubts is damned if he eats, because he eats not of faith: for whatsoever is not of faith is sin."

Romans 6:23A

"For the wages of sin is death."

4. Sickness/Disease.

5. Enslavements/Bondage/Captivity.

Without understanding of God's priorities, there is very little or nothing that we can do.

We cannot ignore God's priority/scale of preference/order of events and follow ours and get His ordained, designed and desired results. It's impossible.

If you are His messenger (Isaiah 44:26; Romans 10:13-15; Proverbs 13:17), our duty is First to Give His Word.

Second to Heal Them

Thirdly to Deliver them from their destructions.

To count 1 and jump 2 and go to 3 is wrong.

To jump 1 and 2 and go to 3 (deliverance) is wrong.

To stay on 1 and ignore/avoid 2Nd 3 is absolutely wrong. Beware of such deadly actions.

Give The Living Word First

Heal Them Secondly

Deliver Them from their destructions Thirdly.

That's God's order of priority as the execution of His duties. Preach The Living Word and Heal before you go into proclamation/Deliverance.

God never sent forth His word and left them in their sicknesses/diseases and bondages/enslavements. Instead of saving and not healing them/delivering them, He'll rather Heal and deliver them from their sicknesses and after wards save them.

It's either He forgives/saves, heals them and delivers them at the same time or He'll rather Heal them first and do the remaining later.

God never sends the sick back home with their ills when they come to Him in faith for their healing.

Psalms 103:3-4 (RSV)-Mankind/Unbelievers.

3 "Who forgives all your iniquity, who heals all your diseases,

4 who redeems your life from the Pit, who crowns you with steadfast love and mercy,"

Psalms 107:20 (RSV)- Israel of God/Believers (Old and New Testament).

"He sent forth his word, and healed them, and delivered them from destruction."

From Psalms 107:20, God by Himself made it very clear that He will heal them (first) once they receive His Word. He didn't say, "He sent forth His word and forgave them and healed them and delivered them from their destructions" That means, when God has a choice to make between forgiveness of sins and Healing of the body, His choice is Healing first, then forgiveness of sins (John 5:8-9; 13-14) or He will forgive sins and also heal diseases (Psalms 103:3-4; Matthew 9:2-7; Mark 2:1-12).

God will send His word, and then forgive sins/Heal at the same time. If He wants to postpone either forgiveness of sins or Healing of the body, He will rather choose to Heal (first) and then forgive later/after wards.

Why then is Healing so important to God?

Nobody can pack into a decaying house. Nobody will see a dying man and not try to save his life before finding out what can be done about the cause of the problem or death and then deal with it. You don't see a man at the point of death and begin to ask him what caused his predicament, and then begin to look for what to do to handle the cause of the problem. The first thing to do is to render first aid/healing to resuscitate life and then later deal with the cause. This was what Jesus did in John 5:8-9,13-14. God does the same also, always (Psalms 107:20).

We must do the same. Give The Living Word, Heal and Deliver from sin, poverty, etc.

Read Psalms 107:10-20 and you will see why God acted the way He did-sent forth His word and Healed them and delivered them from their destructions. That is the best way to respond at such times.

Note: Psalms 107:20 is given to the Redeemed Israelites that sinned against God and by their actions incurred God's wrath. Israel was God's Son. So, when Israel sinned, God sent His word forth, and Healed them and delivered them from their destructions. Compare the New Testament Israel (the church) Galatians 6:16; James 5:14-15. It is the same. Read James 5:14-15. God sent forth The Living Word to show them what to do-call for the elders of the church and let them pray over him, anointing him with oil in the name of the Lord, and the prayer of faith will save the sick man, and the Lord will raise him up, and if he has committed sins, he will be forgiven.

God does not forgive his sins before He heals him. He gives the Living Word (which must be received and obeyed) then He heals the sick and finally delivers him from the cause of it by forgiving his sins.

Psalms 107:20 = James 5:14-15. Both are the same forces.

But for unbelievers;

1.The Living Word is sent forth (published).

2.Then they Hear, Believe/accept it.

3.Then He Forgives their iniquities.

4.Then He Heals their diseases.

5.Then He Redeems them from destructions.

6.Then He Crowns them with love/mercy.

7.Then He Satisfies them with good always so that they live long vigorous lives like the eagles serving Him.

For Believers;

Psalms 68:11

"The Lord gives the command; great is the host of those who bore the tidings:"

Psalms 107:20

"He sent forth his word, and healed them, and delivered them from destruction."

James 5:14-15

14 "Is any among you sick? Let him call for the elders of the church, and let them pray over him, anointing him with oil in the name of the Lord;

15 and the prayer of faith will save the sick man, and the Lord will raise him up; and if he has committed sins, he will be forgiven."

Psalms 103:4-5

4 "Who redeems your life from the Pit, who crowns you with steadfast love and mercy,

5 who satisfies you with good as long as you live so that your youth is renewed like the eagle's."

1. The Living Word is sent forth (published).
2. Hears and obeys (call on the Lord, call on the Elders).
3. Healed.
4. Delivered/Raised up-Psalms 107:20; James 5:5.
5. Forgiven of sins-James 5:15.
6. Crowned with love/mercy.
7. Satisfied with good always, forever.

Why Does God Send The Living Word First?

Simply put, God sends The Living Word first to deal with unbelief/lack of faith, ignorance, lack of knowledge and understanding of what HE wants to do and How He wants it done. Once The Living Word has dealt with the fundamental problem of unbelief as a result of lack of knowledge (Psalms 82:5-7), then He goes forth to heal by confirming His word (Mark 16:19-20; Psalms 107:20; James 5:4-5).

Send The Living Word and Heal and Deliver them from their destructions.

CHAPTER 7

THE CAPTAIN'S RESPONSE
TO HIS DYING SLAVE

Luke 7:2-3 (TLB) – (Read full account Luke 7:2-10; Matthew 8:5-13).

2 "The highly prized slave of a Roman army captain was sick and near death.

3 When the captain heard about Jesus, he sent some respected Jewish elders to ask him to come and heal his slave."

The same story is repeated in Matthew 8:5-13 and Luke 7:1-10- why 2Corinthians 13:1.

The Roman Army Captain was not born again. He was not a Jew. He was a wicked alien yet he was unwilling to let his highly prized slave die of his sickness. And he did all within his power to secure healing for his slave.

In Hebrews 2:10(KJV), Jesus is called THE CAPTAIN OF OUR SALVATION.

If a Roman Army Captain sought and secured the healing of his highly prized slave, why then do people (particularly believers) seem to think it something incredible and impossible for the Captain of our Salvation to seek, secure and administer healing to his friends, brethren and fellow sons and daughters of God; kings and priests and fellow heirs (Romans 8:16-17; Galatians 16:6-7).

Hear me: Beyond the desires of the Roman army captain, our

captain-Jesus Christ does not only desire our salvation/healing/soundness but has done all things needful and have secured our eternal salvation and healing by His blood.

Hebrews 9:12

"He entered once for all into the Holy Place, taking not the blood of goats and calves but his own blood, thus securing an eternal redemption."

Zechariah 9:11

"As for you also, because of the blood of my covenant with you, I will set your captives free from the waterless pit."

1Peter 2:24

"Who his own self bare our sins in his own body on the tree, that we, being dead to sins, should live unto righteousness: by whose stripes ye were healed."

Isaiah 53:4-5

4 "Surely he hath borne our griefs, and carried our sorrows: yet we did esteem him stricken, smitten of God, and afflicted.

5 But he was wounded for our transgressions, he was bruised for our iniquities: the chastisement of our peace was upon him; and with his stripes we are healed."

Matthew 8:17

"That it might be fulfilled which was spoken by Esaias the prophet, saying, Himself took our infirmities, and bare our sicknesses."

You are not one bit justified to carry any trace of disease, illness/sickness in your body. Your body is only to house The Living Word, The Holy Spirit, Jesus Christ and God the Father.

Colossians 2:9-10

9 "For in him dwelleth all the fulness of the Godhead bodily.

10 And ye are complete in him, which is the head of all principality and power:"

The fullness of the Godhead is to be housed in your body.

John 14:20-21,23

20 "At that day ye shall know that I am in my Father, and ye in me, and I in you.

21 He that hath my commandments, and keeps them, he it is

that loveth me: and he that loveth me shall be loved of my Father, and I will love him, and will manifest myself to him.

23 Jesus answered and said unto him, If a man love me, he will keep my words: and my Father will love him, and we will come unto him, and make our abode with him."

1Corinthians 3:16

"Know ye not that ye are the temple of God, and that the Spirit of God dwelleth in you?"

1Corinthians 6:19

"What? know ye not that your body is the temple of the Holy Ghost which is in you, which ye have of God, and ye are not your own?"

2Corinthians 6:16

"And what agreement hath the temple of God with idols? for ye are the temple of the living God; as God hath said, I will dwell in them, and walk in them; and I will be their God, and they shall be my people."

John 10:30

"I and my Father are one."

John 15:1-6

1.I am the true vine, and my Father is the husbandman.

2 Every branch in me that beareth not fruit he taketh away: and every branch that beareth fruit, he purges it, that it may bring forth more fruit.

3 Now ye are clean through the word which I have spoken unto you.

4 Abide in me, and I in you. As the branch cannot bear fruit of itself, except it abide in the vine; no more can ye, except ye abide in me.

5 I am the vine, ye are the branches: He that abideth in me, and I in him, the same bringeth forth much fruit: for without me ye can do nothing.

6 If a man abide not in me, he is cast forth as a branch, and is withered; and men gather them, and cast them into the fire, and they are burned."

The above Scriptures shows very clearly you embody the Godhead. Why allow sickness in your body. Your captain doesn't, so why keep it?

Men are wicked. So the Roman Army Captain as a man is categorized as wicked.

Matthew 7:7-11

7 "Ask, and it shall be given you; seek, and ye shall find; knock, and it shall be opened unto you:

8 For every one that asks receiveth; and he that seeks finds; and to him that knocks it shall be opened.

9 Or what man is there of you, whom if his son ask bread, will he give him a stone?

10 Or if he ask a fish, will he give him a serpent?

11 If ye then, being evil, know how to give good gifts unto your children, how much more shall your Father which is in heaven give good things to them that ask him?"

Luke 11:9-13

9 "And I say unto you, Ask, and it shall be given you; seek, and ye shall find; knock, and it shall be opened unto you.

10 For every one that asks receiveth; and he that seeks finds; and to him that knocks it shall be opened.

11 If a son shall ask bread of any of you that is a father, will he give him a stone? or if he ask a fish, will he for a fish give him a serpent?

12 Or if he shall ask an egg, will he offer him a scorpion?

13 If ye then, being evil, know how to give good gifts unto your children: how much more shall your heavenly Father give the Holy Spirit to them that ask him?"

Romans 8:11

"But if the Spirit of him that raised up Jesus from the dead dwell in you, he that raised up Christ from the dead shall also quicken your mortal bodies by his Spirit that dwelleth in you."

Wicked men still give good gifts to their children or dependents. The Roman Army captain did for his slave.

Why won't the Lord Jesus Christ who purposely came as our Healer (Exodus 15:26; 23:25-26; Deuteronomy 7:11-15; Malachi 3:6; Hebrews 13:8; Acts 10:38,etc) and Saviour from sickness, sin,

Satan, etc (Matthew 1:21-23; Luke 4:18-19; Acts 10:38) save, heal and deliver his own?

When we ask him for healing, He never denies us.

Healing is our bread (Mark 7:27). You can't ask for healing and be denied.

When you ask the Father, He won't deny you of The Holy Spirit. (Luke 11:13). And there is no sickness that can stay in your body when the same Holy Spirit and power of God that raised Jesus Christ from the dead dwells in your mortal bodies. (Romans 1:4; Romans 8:11).

You have every right to be healed and live healthy.

John 10:10

"The thief cometh not, but for to steal, and to kill, and to destroy: I am come that they might have life, and that they might have it more abundantly."

1John 3:8

"He that commits sin is of the devil; for the devil sinneth from the beginning. For this purpose, the Son of God was manifested, that he might destroy the works of the devil."

Jesus came purposely to give you life and health and abundance or prosperity in overflowing abundance. He came to destroy all the works of the devil. Why do you think you must keep what He came to destroy and "died and destroyed?"

I want to believe it is sinful to keep what Jesus came and died to destroy and have destroyed. You won't be happy if you pay your children's school fees and your child still goes ahead to allow himself punished with those whose own fees were not paid by their parents. I know you will be mad at him.

Don't make the Lord get "mad" T you for taking for granted all He has paid for on your behalf.

Your healing/salvation have been paid for by the captain of your salvation. Take what belongs to you and be free in Jesus Name.

I am expecting your testimonies.

BECOME A CITIZEN OF HEAVEN TODAY!

Please note, if you are not yet a Citizen of Heaven, but desire to be, this is your opportunity. To be a citizen of Heaven, you must be from above. You must be born of God. You must be born again!

John 3:3-8,12-13

3 Jesus answered and said to him, "Most assuredly, I say to you, unless one is born again, he cannot see the kingdom of God."

4 Nicodemus said to Him, "How can a man be born when he is old? Can he enter a second time into his mother's womb and be born?"

5 Jesus answered, "Most assuredly, I say to you, unless one is born of water and the Spirit, he cannot enter the kingdom of God.

6 "That which is born of the flesh is flesh, and that which is born of the Spirit is spirit.

7 "Do not marvel that I said to you, 'You must be born again.'

8 "The wind blows where it wishes, and you hear the sound of it, but cannot tell where it comes from and where it goes. So is everyone who is born of the Spirit."

12 If I have told you earthly things, and ye believe not, how shall ye believe, if I tell you of heavenly things?

13 And no man hath ascended up to heaven, but he that came down from heaven, even the Son of man which is in heaven.

Jesus says "You must be born again to live and enjoy Heaven-now!" John 3:3,7

No matter your sin(s) and what you may have done, God wants you forgive and restored now!

John 3:13-18

13 "No one has ascended to heaven but He who came down from heaven, that is, the Son of Man who is in heaven.

14 "And as Moses lifted up the serpent in the wilderness, even so must the Son of Man be lifted up,

15 "that whoever believes in Him should not perish but have eternal life.

16 "For God so loved the world that He gave His only begotten Son, that whoever believes in Him should not perish but have everlasting life.

17 "For God did not send His Son into the world to condemn the world, but that the world through Him might be saved.

18 "He who believes in Him is not condemned; but he who does not believe is condemned already, because he has not believed in the name of the only begotten Son of God.

Remember God gives the power to become His son to everyone that receives Jesus as The Christ, The Son of The Living God or believe in His Name. John 1:12

Remember God Himself dwells in everyone who believes and confesses that Jesus is The Christ, The Son of The Living God. 1John 5:1, 4-5;1John 4:4,15

Remember God did not send His Son into the world to condemn the world but that through Him, the world might be saved. John 3:17

Beloved, AS the Father sent Jesus The Christ, even so has The Lord Jesus Christ sent me so that everyone who will believe and receive me as His Ambassador will be saved, healed, delivered and restored. The Lord said to me: As the Father sent Me, even so have I sent you! John 17:18; John 20:21

The Lord said to Me: Verily, verily I say to you, whoever receives you receives me, and whoever receives me receives the Father who sent me. John 13:20.

The Lord said to Me: Whoever rejects you rejects me, and whoever rejects Me rejects The Father who sent Me. Luke 10:16

The Lord said to Me: Behold I give unto you power to tread upon serpents and scorpions and over all the power of the enemy and nothing shall by any means hurt you. Luke 10:19

The Lord said to Me: Behold, I send in the midst of many peoples, like dew from the LORD, like showers on the grass, that tarry for no man nor wait for the sons of men. Behold, you shall be among the Gentiles, In the midst of many peoples, like a lion among the beasts of the forest, like a young lion among flocks of sheep, Who, if he passes through, both treads down and tears in pieces, and none can deliver. Your hand shall be lifted against your adversaries, and all your enemies shall be cut off. Micah 5:7-9

The Lord said to Me: You will be like the dew to all My people and creation; You shall grow like the lily, and lengthen Your roots like Lebanon. Your branches shall spread; Your beauty shall be like an olive tree, And Your fragrance like Lebanon. Those who dwell under Your shadow shall return; They shall be revived like grain, and grow like a vine. Their scent shall be like the wine of Lebanon. Hosea 14:5-7

Beloved, there is no justifiable reason under Heaven why you should ever go through ANYTHING that is not in Heaven now!

Beloved there is no justifiable reason why you should not have NOW the best God has fully paid for and credited to your personal account!

Hear Me: All things are ready. And all things are yours! What are you still waiting for? All you need to do is to believe that Jesus is the Christ, The Son of The Living God. And He sent Me to bring this Goodnews to you.

Your struggles can come to an end today. You can be enrolled into Heaven's citizenship right now. You can begin a new life today and enjoy all that is available in Heaven from this day forward. The Lord Jesus Christ who sent me confirms with undeniable proof that He is ALIVE today in the lives of those who hear my words and believes in Him [The Lord Jesus Christ] who sent me.

Jesus is alive today and the only way to prove it is for Him to do what He did before in your life today. He sent me and will prove to you that this is not a made-up story written to impress you, but His ordained will made available to make you are created to be!

The choice is yours! Rise and take what belong to you and enter your rest!

Peace now and always in Jesus Almighty Name!

Amen!!!

If You are not certain that You are Born Again as you are certain of your name, or You were once saved but went astray again, living and doing as you pleased, then say this Prayer aloud now for you to become a citizen of Heaven:

PRAYER FOR SALVATION AND RESTORATION TO HEAVEN'S CITIZENSHIP!

Dear Heavenly Father, I return to you by Faith. I am sorry for my sins. I believe in my heart that Jesus is The Christ and that He died for my sins and rose from the dead on the third day, according to Scripture, for my justification. I confess that Jesus Christ is LORD and I accept Him now as my Saviour. I believe my sins are wiped away.

I call upon The Name of The LORD for my total Healing, Liberty and Restoration.

I ask for the Gift of Your Holy Spirit, Power and Grace to follow and serve You from this day forward. And I Thank You Abba Father for doing far beyond all I have asked and can ever imagine in Jesus Name. Amen!

I Now Declare That I Am A Child of God Forever! There's no going back.

Now that you have become a Citizen of Heaven, you need to upgrade by signing up to serve as an Ambassador for Christ. That is where your security and relevance lie. There is no job in this world that can be compared to serving as The Ambassador of The King of kings and Lord of lords. The benefits are amazing. You cannot do a better or more honourable job.

You can Enlist now and become a Partner or a Member of

our Totally Empowered Ambassadors on Mission (TEAM) and see what Our Risen Lord and King Jesus Christ will transform your life into and do in, for and through you from this day as you believe and obey His Word!

I can't wait to hear from you because I believe you have been blessed and helped immensely reading this Book as much as I am writing it! I am praying for you.

ABOUT THE AUTHOR

Amb. Promise Ogbonna

Amb Promise Ogbonna is the President of Christ's Ambassadors Living Mission International Inc. aka Jesus Mission Headquarters, an all-encompassing network of ministries with a mandate focus to Preach The Everlasting Gospel to all, Stop anything after man's destruction, Bring Healing, Liberty and Restoration to all, Make ALL Christ's Ambassadors and Make Heaven-Now a Reality for All.

He is the Publisher of ONTOP Life Publishers Company with a commission to Publish the Everlasting Gospel and Bring God's Wisdom-solutions for every problem and need of mankind.

He represents The Lord Jesus Christ and serves Him as His Ambassador!

He is married and blessed with children.

OTHER BOOKS BY AMB PROMISE OGBONNA

1. The Nothingness of Satan
2. You Can Make a Fresh Start and Rule Your World
3. Restoring The Forgotten Dignity of Woman
4. Christ's Ambassadors: Re-Emergence of Rulers in
5. Why Prophet Elisha Died Sick and how to Avoid it
6. You Can Choose When to Die
7. You Shall Live and Not Die
8. Why Christians Die Sick
9. 7 Keys to Undeniable Healing
10. 8 Decisive Hours That Will Take You To The Topmost
11. Activating God's Medicine For Your Healing
12. God Cannot Fail To Heal You
13. Healing Is Your Legal Right
14. God's Final Solution to The Problem of The Black Race
15. Understanding God's Secret to Winning Life's Battles
16. 100 Years Is Minimum
17. How to Raise The Dead
18. Manifesting as Signs and Wonders: Unlocking The Unstoppable You Regardless of Where You are Now!
19. 40 Pitfalls to Avoid in Life – Mastering The Art of Living Successfully.
20. Wisdom Seeds to Greatness In Life – Inspiring Seed-Thoughts on Being Your Best
21. God's Medicine for Incurable Diseases
22. Ambassador Promise: Jesus Christ's Official Ambassador and T. L. Osborn's Successor on Earth Today! Appearance and En-

counters with The Lord Jesus Christ, Mantles of Notable Servants of God Received and The 9 Mandates.

23. Simple Faith for Supernatural Success
24. God's Final Message to The Poor
25. Understanding The Gospel to The Poor
26. Faith That Attracts God's Attention and Results
27. God's Quickest Way to Your Prosperity and Restoration
28. Faith for Healing
29. Unveiling God's Master Keys to Your Dominion Against All Odds
30. Operating the Faith that Pleases God
31. 4 Kinds of People The Lord Will Heal
32. Appropriating Your Healing

UPCOMING BOOKS BY AMB PROMISE OGBONNA

1. Enforcing Kingdom Wealth Transfer
2. God's Final Word on Tithes, Tithing and Offerings
3. Creating Heaven Out of Your Ruined World
4. How to Attract God's Blessing on Your Business and Career
5. How to Make Your Faith Work
6. God's Master Key to Your Dominion
7. Wisdom Keys To God's Recovery Plan
8. Jesus Christ's Teaching on Provoking Our Covenant Heritage of Prosperity
9. Why People Fail in Life –Secrets to Success without Stress

Please visit your favorite eBook retailer to discover other books by Amb Promise Ogbonna.

CONNECT WITH AMB PROMISE OGBONNA

I appreciate you reading my book. Here are my links and Social Coordinates

Send Amb Promise Ogbonna a mail at:

Visit Amb. Promise Ogbonna's Website:

Subscribe to Amb Promise Ogbonna's videos at:

Follow Amb Promise Ogbonna on Twitter:

Friend Amb Promise Ogbonna on Facebook:

Connect with Amb Promise Ogbonna on LinkedIn:

Read Amb Promise Ogbonna's Story at Wattpad:

Subscribe to Amb Promise Ogbonna's Blog at:

Follow Amb Promise Ogbonna on Instagram:

Subscribe to Amb. Promise Ogbonna's HEAVENow You Tube Channel:

Read Amb Promise Ogbonna's Smashwords Interview at

Read Amb Promise Ogbonna's Author Profile at Smashwords:

Follow Amb Promise Ogbonna at Amazon:

Connect with Amb Promise Ogbonna on Pinterest:

Read Amb. Promise Ogbonna books at Okada Books:

Get Access to all the Books of Amb Promise Ogbonna at Books2Read Universal Book Link:

JOIN AMB. PROMISE OGBONNA IN HEAVENOW SERVICES

Worship with Ambassador Promise in Christ's Ambassadors Heaven-Now Services at:

Christ's Ambassadors Living Mission International [Jesus Mission Headquarters]

24 Independence Street, Behind O'Mark Schools by O'Mark Bus Stop, LASU Road, Igando Lagos

Wednesdays: 12:00-1:00pm. Hour of EmPowerment for All [Online]

Saturdays: 8:00-9:00am. Hour of Healing for All

Sundays: 8:00-9:00am. Hour of Liberty and Restoration for All

Sundays: 9:00-10:00am. Hour of Kingdom Wealth Transfer for All

Last Friday Night Monthly: 10pm. Night of Restorations for All

Ambassadors International Bible Institute: Runs Online and Offline Courses to Make Christ's Ambassadors and Make Heaven Now a reality for all. Enroll today!

HEAVENow…Making Heaven now a Reality for ALL!

OUR HEALING PRODUCTS

We are on a Mission to Bring Healing to the sick no matter their sicknesses or diseases and Restore Health, Wealth and Peace to ALL! Here are some of our Products and Services we run to Bring Healing to the sick worldwide!

1. All-Purpose Divine Healing Medicine
2. Healing Messages – Podcasts, CD, MP3 and DVD
3. Healing Books
4. Healing Leaves Magazine
5. Healing Anointing Oil
6. Healing Mantles and Clothes
7. Healing Materials
8. Healing Elixir for incurable diseases
9. Healing Songs
10. Healing Homes
11. Health Centers
12. Healing Balm

Call us today for all of your Healing needs! We are here to SERVE YOU!

OUR SPECIAL SERVICES

We Offer the following services to Churches, Ministries, Corporate Bodies, Businesses, Communities, Groups, International Bodies, NGO's, Governments, States and Nations.

1. Healing Seminars
2. Healing School
3. Healing Teams
4. Healing Outreaches and Explosions
5. World Healing Conferences
6. Health and Wealth Trainings
7. Heaven-Now Campaigns
8. Kingdom Wealth Transfer Seminars
9. God's FASTEST Prosperity Recovery Seminars
10. Heaven's Business School
11. Time and Stress Management Training
12. Leadership Responsibility Development Training

Our Services are geared towards making every person fit spirit, soul and body so that they can be empowered to deliver results competently, effectively and efficiently.

For Bookings Contact us today!